GET THAT SOUND SLEEP

Helpful Tips to have a sound sleep

Florence Martha

Table of contents

Introduction

We all tend to suffer from Insomnia at a point in life. It can be triggered by stressful periods in our careers, personal crises, fears about an upcoming event, or financial worries that can keep us awake and restless.

Guilt or grief is another culprit.

Whatever the reason for your tossing and turning, you know what it feels like to get out of bed in the morning. You are running out of energy. Your body is in pain and your brain is foggy. You feel irritable and grumpy. Your sleepless nights will reflect throughout your day – and not for the better.

Over time, sleep problems can become extremely debilitating. Prolonged sleep deprivation will negatively impact your career, social life, and personal relationships. Sometimes they can test your sanity.

For some people, insomnia is a chronic problem. For others, it comes and goes sometimes. While for most people, insomnia can be closely related to the quality or duration of sleep. Lack of sleep can really harm our minds and physical health. This can lead to serious problems like depression, high blood pressure, and loss of control of the hormonal system. This puts our bodies at higher risk of chronic diseases and accelerates the aging process.

Since reading this book, you may be having trouble sleeping and want to do something about it. You may have tried countless remedies (glass of warm milk before bed or counting sheep). You may have resorted to prescription drugs, adding to the addiction risk to your problem. However, nothing seems to work. Then, are you doomed to live with your sleep problems for the rest of your life?

Absolutely not.

Biohacking is the solution to the problem of sleep deprivation once and for all. It's completely safe, easy, relatively free, and guaranteed to get you through your sleep problems. The biohacking tools you're about to explore will make it easy to modify and adjust your individual sleep patterns. They will help you develop a plan that leads to specific changes to optimize your sleep and improve your overall health and well-being.

Incorporating these biohacking techniques into your lifestyle will make a lasting change, allowing you to confidently get a healthy night's sleep every time.

Chapter 1: What is Biohacking

Do you eat more fish oil to improve your brain health? Do you use essential oils to relieve stress and improve your mood? Maybe you follow a diet rich in antioxidants or exercise regularly to improve your heart health. If so, then you are already a biohacker! In fact, most of us are biohackers in one form or another without even knowing it.

What is biohacking? Biohacking is the process of modifying your lifestyle habits in order to "hack" your body's biological functions and achieve positive changes in health.

• Biohacking is simply "do it yourself" biology. Simple changes (such as diet, exercise, and sleep patterns) are made to improve health, protect against disease, and correct problems like sleep deprivation.

• This is a relatively new method and although it is based on biology, it is not considered a science in itself. However, its potential can be huge. Field studies are underway and the results are promising. Biohacking has been shown to have a major impact on many areas of physical and mental health.

• Biohacking is an experimental process because not all body cycles and rhythms are created equal. Some people may react to certain "hacks" while others may not. So it's all about trying different hacks to find the one that works best for you. It is by no means meant to experiment with your body in a way that can be harmful. These tools are completely safe to use and see which – if not all – improves your sleep.

• Leading experts in the field of biohacking are Dave Asprey and Ben Greenfield. They test themselves, develop new products and tips in the field of nutrition and fitness and share them with the world.

There are three types of biological attacks:

1.Nutrigenomics deals with nutrition, stress management, and penetrating your environment, such as sound and light.

2. DIYBIO or DIY bio. This is where amateur scientists conduct biohacking experiments and share the results with like-minded people. The

goal is to prove that an ordinary person can become a successful biohacker.

3. Biohacking Grinder focuses on technologies such as implants and the addition of chemicals to attack the body's biology. This is absolutely NOT recommended as the risks may outweigh the benefits. Best leave that to the complete fanatics.

What should you focus on? Sleep scientists tell us the hours don't matter. The quality of your sleep is essential to your physical and mental health.

Many people sleep 7-8 hours a night but still wake up tired and tossing and turning. This is because their sleep quality is poor. They are unable to enter a state of deep sleep that relaxes and rejuvenates the body. Quality sleep means waking up full of energy and vitality, no matter how many hours you sleep. This should be your main goal; Not only sleepy but also sleep well.

We can use a number of safe and natural biohacking techniques to improve the overall quality of sleep. The following chapters will discuss some of the most popular and successful sleep tricks. These will help you:

• Overcoming insomnia

• Fall asleep faster

• Improve sleep time

• Improve sleep quality

• For deep sleep, restore health

A few so called specialists claim that biohacking requires different contraptions and complex estimations to screen brain waves and other reactions. Honestly, this is completely unnecessary.

Always remember that no one understands your body better than you. You may know what works best for you by how you are feeling. You will be able to measure the results based on the improvement in your sleep.

You may find that you love biohacking so much that you want to dig deeper. As your knowledge and skills increase, you may want to try measuring gadgets and tools. But for now, let's keep it simple.

Chapter 2: Stopping the use of blue light

Science says that light from the blue side of the spectrum interferes with the brain's production of melatonin, the hormone that controls sleep and wakefulness. Exposure to blue light, especially in the evening, can significantly disrupt sleep.

Blue light includes light coming in through windows, as well as light from traditional and LED bulbs. Digital screens such as PCs, laptops, tablets and TV screens also emit large amounts of blue light.

This hack is easy. The quickest and most effective way to improve your sleep is to block all light from your bedroom.

There are several ways to do this.

• Use blackout curtains to completely block the sun. This is especially useful when:

People who wake up late or sleep during the day on night shifts.

• If you absolutely cannot sleep in a completely dark room, a low-intensity amber nightlight is fine. These types of bulbs do not emit blue light. The hallway leading to the restrooms can also be dimmed with amber lighting. This will help you quickly fall asleep again when you return to bed.

• Invest in a sleep mask that filters out blue light. However, keep in mind that blue light is absorbed throughout the body through the skin. If this method doesn't work, try blackout curtains. • Make sure the lighting in your home is suitable for sleeping. Our bodies start producing melatonin a few hours before we go to bed, causing drowsiness. But too much lighting in your home can inhibit melatonin production, not just on your TV or computer screen. Make sure your home is dimly lit (amber or red and yellow spectrum lighting works best) and don't watch TV or sit in front of your computer right before bed.

That's because when the skin absorbs blue light, it starts producing cortisol, a hormone that counteracts the effects of melatonin, which increases alertness and induces sleep.

• Wear amber glasses for the last 3-4 hours of the day. Here's another simple hack to help with "melatonin production in the dark". This terminology refers to the production of melatonin in the evening. Amber glasses, glasses with yellow or orange lenses, are very inexpensive, but may be the best choice for a better night's sleep. They are also available on Amazon and elsewhere on the internet in a variety of designs. In the evening, it recognizes and drives away blue light sources in its surroundings. This hack will improve your sleep in just a few days and you should see immediate results.

Chapter 3: Try Sleep Apps

The sleep app is scientifically designed to help you get a good night's sleep. We recommend doing this when biohacking, as they are easy to use and contain diverse features that you can choose and experiment with.

These are specially designed to create a relaxing experience that calms your brain waves and induces restful sleep. Ideally, it helps maintain a restful sleep throughout the night.

Sleep apps usually offer soothing audio recordings that calm the brain and encourage sleep. These include gentle rain sounds, ocean waves, wind blowing through trees, and other natural sounds. Some apps offer guided meditations, white noise, and various ambient sounds.

Some apps offer a wide range of relaxing classical and contemporary music, so there is something for every taste and taste. It's fun to experiment with these different sounds and find the one that works best to disrupt sleep.

Other features include:

• Dashboard showing sleep patterns and sleep quality percentages. There are also apps that can measure snoring.

• If you have an artistic flair, you can use apps like Recolor to create brain-relaxing artwork. A special color palette is provided that is designed to reduce anxiety and promote sleep.

• Many apps contain hypnotic tracks to calm and relax your brain.

• Some include alarms to help you sync short naps throughout the day. . Most sleep apps are free for both Android and iPhone. Prices for products with more advanced features range from $3 to $9.99.

Helpful hints:

White noise in general is a good sleep inducer, and many studies have backed this up. It stabilizes your brain waves and helps you sleep soundly all night. If you don't want to use a sleep app, you can easily access white noise with a fan. Works equally well with ceiling fans and regular fans. Just leave it on overnight. The sound lulls you to sleep, and the steady buzzing sound will help you sleep soundly all night.

Try some free apps first. If you enjoy using it and get good results, that's great. Otherwise you are not wasting your money.

Chapter 4: Try stepping out in the sun

In this case, the blue light from the sun can actually help you sleep better. As we discussed in Chapter 1, we should avoid blue light in the evening. However, blue light exposure during the day is another matter, so don't confuse it.

When exposed to sunlight, our bodies send signals to the pituitary gland and hypothalamus to help maintain circadian rhythms. The circadian rhythm is simply our body's internal clock. For good quality sleep, it is important to maintain a balanced and stable sleep. Our circadian rhythm also regulates many important hormones, including melatonin. As mentioned earlier, melatonin is essential for sleep. It also helps with depression, which can affect sleep quality.

It works like this:

The Exposure to daylight amid the day increments "low-light melatonin production," which starts after nightfall. Spending time in the sun increases melatonin production even in dim light, preparing your body for restful sleep. This is one of the easiest sleep hacks and it's completely free. It can be as simple as taking a walk in the park on your lunch break or sipping a smoothie at a sidewalk cafe. No matter how busy your life is, there are still plenty of ways to catch sin.

How much time should you actually spend under the sun? Ideally at least 15-20 minutes a day. Of course, this also depends on several factors such as the climate you live in, the season, the time of day, skin sensitivity, and how much skin you expose. Sitting near a bright window is another way to expose your skin to blue light during the day, according to research. A great technique for rainy days or when it's too cold to go outside.

Use light therapy box

If regular sun exposure is difficult, a light therapy box can be a good option. A device that emits blue wavelength light. Designed to balance your circadian rhythms. Just like solar radiation.

Place the crate a few feet away from you, but don't look directly at it. It is recommended to place it on the periphery of the field of view. Expose to light for 15-30 minutes. Reveal as much skin as possible during the session. Ideally, you should do this at the same time each day to maintain your circadian rhythm.

Please. Another super easy and hassle free sleep hack.

Chapter 5: Sleep-Friendly Food Tricks

We all love food, and luckily this eating trick includes foods that everyone loves. This trick allows you to unleash your creativity and make dishes that are not only delicious, but also help you sleep like a baby!

The following is a list of sleep-friendly foods that have been proven to be highly beneficial for sleep. Add them to your diet, particularly at dinnertime and be astounded at how the quality of your sleep progresses.

- Kiwi

- Fatty fish (salmon, tuna, halibut, mackerel)

- Cherries

- Poultry

- Avocadoes

- Leafy greens, especially spinach

- Nuts, especially pistachios, almonds, and walnuts

- Cheese

- Chamomile tea

- Starchy foods (potatoes, yams, plantains)

- Peanut butter

- Bananas

- Oatmeal and cereal

These nourishments contain tryptophan, an amino corrosive that produces serotonin (a hormone the soothes stress, advances calmness and elevates the temperament). They also contain the all-important melatonin. Regular consumption of these foods promotes what scientists call "sleep hygiene." Sleep hygiene is the eating habits you adopt to promote sleep, especially before you go to bed.

The best part is that not only are the above foods popular with many, they can be combined into salads, desserts, casseroles, or eaten alone on a daily basis. Make a habit of eating at least one or two at every meal, especially at dinner. A handful of nuts, a small bowl of oatmeal, or a banana also make great bedtime snacks. We think you'll agree that practicing food hygiene is an easy and fun way to do it. So get creative! Experiment with sleep-friendly foods to find the best sleep hacks for your body.

Do not disturb sleep by eating foods such as:

• Coffee, sodas, and energy drinks are all high in caffeine (soft drinks other than cola also contain caffeine).

• chocolate

• Spicy food and chillies

• peppermint

• Alcohol (While alcohol can make you temporarily drowsy, it is actually a serious sleep disruptor. Alcoholic beverages make it difficult for your brain to enter the deep sleep cycles necessary for a good night's sleep.)

• High-fat foods.

• Salty food.

• Foods that contain a lot of water, such as watermelon and cantaloupe. You don't want to disturb your sleep by going to the bathroom too often.

That doesn't mean you should permanently eliminate these foods from your diet. Personally, I can't work without my morning coffee. Limit your sleep to the hours of the day to prepare your body for restful sleep.

If you feel like eating hamburgers and potato chips, eat them for lunch. Try to avoid sleep-disrupting foods after noon.

Chapter 6: Acupressure Mat Trick

This is a regular foam mattress, with a pocke
It is embedded with plastic discs wit
protruding ends. These mats are said to b
modeled the nail bed used by meditator
during meditation – ouch! But don't worry;
reflexology mat is not nearly as difficult! It i
similar to a massage chair or acupressur
machine but at a fraction of the cost.

They are available online. Acupressure mat
are actually last very long and are easil
washable. How does acupressure mat work?

A typical mat has more than 800 "massage points" or spikes that help massage deep into your body. They help relax tense muscles, relieve pain, and promote restful sleep.

Millions of users report an immediate improvement in sleep quality, especially when they use it at night.

• The reflexology mat also works as a talisman to relieve back, neck and joint pain. If you suffer from these conditions in addition to lack of sleep, you'll get a double benefit.

• It improves metabolism and digestion, so it is truly a "hollow potion" for overall health and well-being.

• It improves blood circulation, which also promotes good sleep.

How to use acupressure mat?

Carpets are versatile and can be used on your couch, couch, bed or floor. It's light enough to carry to anyplace(beach and parks included) All you have to do is lie on it for at least 2-30 minutes a day or as long as you like. You can use it twice a day if you have time, once in the morning and then in the evening. It is totally secure and has no side impacts.

• Schedule time each day to enjoy a relaxing session, just as you would with a massage therapist.

• The first 3-5 minutes will be a bit painful but as you get used to it you will feel comfortable and enjoy the feeling. It has been described by users as "pure happiness".

• For intense massage, it is recommended to use on the floor. Some people love it but others find it too annoying. Experiment with different surfaces and see which works best for you.

• The more skin exposed to the mat, the greater the benefit. You may want to wear a bathing suit or even get completely naked if your privacy is guaranteed. • If you enjoy yoga or meditation, you can practice on the mat to relieve stress and relax.

Limitations

There are usually no restrictions on gender or even age.

There are only three exceptions:

• If you are pregnant

• If you have a rash

- If you have any cuts, wounds or burns on your skin.

Chapter 7: Use of Binaural Beats and Music Therapy

Binaural beats are auditory sounds that influence brain waves. The frequency of your heartbeat changes your brainwaves to produce specific results. Binaural beats are used to improve creativity, concentration and sleep.

How do binaural beats work?

- Good stereo headphones are required because each ear hears different frequencies. There are headphones on the market specifically designed for binaural beats, but any good quality pair will work just as well.

• The frequency of each tone must be less than 30 Hz to be effective. This allows him to hear two different beats together as one tone.

• The brain interprets the two beats as one coherent tone frequency. This is called frequency following response. Then, adjust the wave according to this sound.

• Binaural beats are designed using specific algorithms that hack your brain to specific frequencies. Our brain uses different frequencies when performing tasks. For example, we use delta and theta waves for sleep. They are associated with relaxation, rest and deep sleep. The binaural beats you hear hack your brain to produce these brain waves.

If you think binaural beats are some kind of weird alien music, you're dead wrong. They are incredibly gentle, fantastic and beautiful. You will experience calm, blissful thoughts as you fall into a peaceful sleep.

If you like it, you can invest in a very affordable audio track pack or subscription. Note that you need really good headphones to really take advantage of this hack.

Music therapy

If nature sounds and binaural beats aren't your thing, there are other options. Music therapy is the perfect hack for music lovers. Music therapy, or the utilisation of alleviating music, has been logically proven to improve sleep and relaxation . Great for reducing physical stress that can cause sleep disturbances. Additionally, music therapy has been shown to balance circadian rhythms.

How does it work?

When soothing music waves connect with our brain waves, we relax and begin to fall asleep. Over time, the brain associates this type of music with rest and sleep. You will quickly learn how to relax and have no trouble falling asleep. What does "comfortable" music mean?

Loud, fast music like hard rock and rap alerts the brain and wakes it up. Soothing music is the opposite. It's slow with soft beats and rhythms. Studies show that the best music to help you fall asleep is:

• Classical music such as sonatas and piano pieces. Favorite song is Beethoven's Moonlight Sonata

• Softlock. If you're a rock lover, save hard rock for the day. Instead, listen to your favorite soft rock track before bed. These should be tracks that focus on the melody and lyrics rather than the beat.

• Ambient music. This includes slow to medium beat instrumentals. You can even find instrumental versions of your favorite songs. One of his most popular hotels is the Hotel California.

• Hymns. A good choice for those with more religious or spiritual tendencies. Again, it's a good idea to try out these different audio therapies. You may find that some genres work better for you, even if they aren't necessarily your favorite genres. Who knows? You may not be religious, but find hymns helpful.

Chapter 8: The science of Aromatherapy

any people view aromatherapy with
kepticism. They consider it a fad or something
sed by meditation and spiritual fanatics.

ut science has shown that the scent of
ssential oils affects our brains in different
ays. They can calm anxiety, improve mood,

and inspire optimism. More importantly, they are powerful anti-insomnia agents. How to use essential oils

Use a diffuser. The best way to use essential oils is to inhale the aroma. Indeed, the olfactory nerves of our nose are directly connected to the brain. The scent of the essential oil quickly travels to the brain, activating sleep-promoting hormones. You also get the added benefit of having your room and home filled with a beautiful fragrance. Diffusers are very cheap and can be purchased almost anywhere that sells essential oils. A cotton pad soaked in essential oils and placed near your bed is also a good choice.

Essential oils are 100% safe to use when diffused. Children and pets will not be harmed by inhaling the fragrance. In fact, your kids, your car and your dog will get better quality sleep too!

Use essential oils in the bath. A few drops of essential oils in a warm bath will create a pleasant and relaxing experience. The fragrance of the oil and the warm water will work together to put you within the ideal temperament for sleep.

Note:

Take a hot shower an hour before bed, not just before. Hot water stimulates circulation for a while, which will keep you awake.

Spray bed linens with essential oils. Use a spray bottle to lightly spray bed sheets and pillowcases. Thus, will create a fragrant sleeping paradise that lasts all night.

Below is a list of essential oils recommended for sleep problems.

- Chamomile essential oil. It is a natural sedative that is extremely easy to fall asleep.

- Marjoram essential oil. Natural antidepressants and anxiolytics help you sleep better.

- Sage essential oil. It is also a very calming and natural sedative.

- Frankincense essential oil. It is hailed as a miracle oil due to its many therapeutic properties. As a sleep aid, it lowers your body temperature to the optimum level needed for quality sleep. It also clears the nasal passages, allowing you to breathe deeply while you sleep.

- Ylang ylang essential oil. Lowers blood pressure and stimulates feelings of tranquility and peace.

- Lavender oil. This oil has been used for centuries to calm and relax. In addition to its wonderful scent, lavender is also a great sleep aid. It promotes REM sleep. This is a deep sleep in which the heart rate slows down and the muscles relax completely. It's the best quality sleep you can get.

• Essential oils of orange, rose. When combined, these two oils form a powerful sedative that smells delicious.

• Valerian essential oil. The scent of this oil will help you sleep through the night. It also helps to relax the body and promotes feelings of peace and happiness.

• Bergamot essential oil. Promotes better sleep by lowering heart rate and blood pressure. It also gives you the added benefit of reducing anxiety.

At the other end of the spectrum are oils that promote energy and alertness. Some of them include rosemary, mint, grapefruit, lemon, and cypress. Products containing these ingredients can also make you sleepless, so avoid using them at night. Instead of helping you relax, they energize you. However, they are great tricks to use in the morning, especially on busy days when you start to feel exhausted.

Chapter 9: Helpful Tips for Sleep

Here are some additional biohacking tips that make sense. In fact, you probably already use them. In addition to the more specific tricks discussed here, these little extra tweaks will give you that extra advantage.

Exercise regularly. Having a regular exercise routine improves overall health and a healthy body is important for quality sleep. Exercise doesn't have to be an aerobics class or a workout. Cycling, swimming, and walking in nature are equally healthy. Just make sure you exercise your body regularly.

Remember that exercising before bed is not a good idea as it will give you energy.

Relax before going to bed. Set aside an hour for a relaxing activity before bed. Read a book, meditate if you're interested, or spend some quiet time chatting with your partner.

Avoid stressful activities that will keep you awake for hours. If you're nervous or easily scared, don't watch horror movies. Don't start an argument with your spouse about finances. Avoid putting yourself in a situation that could cause you stress.

A quiet environment promotes good sleep. If family members are standing, ask them to reduce the noise. Turn off your cell phone if possible. Repair any noisy equipment such as air conditioners or boilers. Check for extra noises that may disturb sleep. If you are a light sleeper, this is doubly important.

A good way to eliminate noise is to play soft music or nature sounds in your bedroom throughout the night.

Buy the best quality essential oils. Not all essential oils are created equal. For maximum benefit, buy only the best quality. They must be labeled 100% pure or 1oo% organic.

Invest in a top-quality mattress. Your mattress is not something you want to save on. This is the "basis" that will make biological attack truly optimal. You may not know it, but most mattresses are stuffed with highly toxic materials. Flame retardants in particular are extremely harmful to health as well as sleep quality. These toxins can take years to clear, and in the meantime, you're breathing them in!

A 100% natural or organic mattress is one of the smartest investments you can make. Do your due diligence and take the time to shop around and look at different brands. It will be expensive, but look at it this way:

Don't you value your health more? Wi-Fi Switch: Wi-Fi waves can interfere with your brain waves during sleep. Just turn it off and generally don't leave any router in your room.

Make sure your bedroom temperature is ideal for sleep. The best temperature for optimal sleep is between 60 and 67 degrees F. As you fall asleep, your body temperature drops, so keeping your bedroom cool helps with this process. Keep your room at this temperature as much as possible, try to wear socks and have a hot water bottle ready when you get cold.

Take a sleep-promoting supplement. Natural supplements are completely different from sleeping pills because they are completely natural and have no side effects. They can be helpful if your body lacks certain sleep-promoting vitamins and minerals. Vitamin B-5, vitamin B12, vitamin D and magnesium, iron, calcium and vitamin E are important for stabilizing circadian rhythms. You can buy them over-the-counter to improve your sleep.

Chapter 10: The summary

So what can we learn from all these?

We have seen how to use biohacking to optimize sleep.

We have seen that sleep hacking requires no advanced scientific knowledge or complicated equipment.

Biohacking is a series of small lifestyle changes that help your body function better.

Biohacking is simple and inexpensive. It's a completely natural way to promote sleep.

So, how do you get started using the biohacks discussed here? Which is the best to start with? Can we use them all together? How to set up the perfect biological attack plan? If you're new to biohacking, it's normal to feel a bit overwhelmed. The key is to start small. Think of biohacking as a toolkit. All the techniques discussed here are different tools in this toolkit. First, you need to customize these tools to suit your needs. Then you need to adjust them to get the best results.

For example, say you want to start with binaural beats. Download a few and use them for some nights. Note any change in your sleep and rate it on a scale of 1 to 1o. 1 will be a noticeable improvement and 1o will not. Then, try listening to music or nature sounds and see if that helps you sleep better. Record and evaluate your findings. Play with different audio tracks until you choose the hearing hack that works best for you. Then switch to a new tool and repeat the process.

If you choose to use a reflexology mat, try it on different surfaces and see how it feels. If you find it too annoying, throw it away and move on to another hack, and so on.

Remember that there is no best or worst sleeping trick. Rule of thumb is what works best for you.

Suggest:

• Start with one or two tips that impress you the most. Provide yourself a week or two to test and see what comes about after.. • Incorporate good sleep tips into your daily routine. Hone them frequently until they end up becoming a habit.

• Switch to another hack and repeat the process.

• I recommend starting with sleep eating tips. This is the simplest way and requires nothing more than consuming the foods listed here. •

Practice makes perfect! You may notice immediate results or a gradual improvement in your sleep over days or weeks. Don't give up too quickly.

• However, biohacking tools do not always yield immediate results. Your brain needs time to adapt to the new stimuli you teach it. Patience and practice are key here. Allow two weeks as a timeframe for each hack to start working before moving on to the new one. Miss:

Biohacking is an experimental process. It's a process of trial and error to discover what works best for your sleeping pattern.

Conclusion

Sleep deprivation is a problem that can paralyze your life. It can prevent you from reaching peak performance. It can affect both your mental and physical health tremendously. It can hurt relationships. More importantly, it prevents you from enjoying life. Biohacking has been scientifically proven to improve sleep quality. There's nothing to lose and a lot to gain by applying these tricks to your routine.

Finally, biohacking is fun! Once you get the hang of it, you'll want to tap into other areas of your life like academic and sports achievements, weight loss, and even improving relationships with others. With biohacking, the sky really is the limit.